MOMENTS WITH ONESELF SERIES: 14

STRESS-FREE LIVING

SWAMI DAYANANDA SARASWATI
ARSHA VIDYA

ARSHA VIDYA
RESEARCH AND PUBLICATION TRUST
CHENNAI

Published by :
Arsha Vidya Research and Publication Trust
4 ' Sri Nidhi ' Apts 3rd Floor
Sir Desika Road Mylapore
Chennai 600 004 INDIA
Tel : 044 2499 7023
Telefax : 2499 7131
Email : avrandpt@gmail.com
Website: www.avrpt.com

ISBN : 978-81-906059-3-9

First Edition :	October	2008	Copies : 1000
1st Reprint :	May	2009	Copies : 2000
2nd Reprint :	January	2010	Copies : 2000
3rd Reprint :	March	2011	Copies : 1000
4th Reprint :	May	2012	Copies : 1000

Design & layout :
Graaphic Design

Printed at :
Sudarsan Graphics
27, Neelakanta Mehta Street
T. Nagar, Chennai 600 017
Email : info@sudarsan.com

Contents

Key to Transliteration and Pronunciation of Sanskrit Letters

Sanskrit is a highly phonetic language and hence accuracy in articulation of the letters is important. For those unfamiliar with the *Devanāgari* script, the international transliteration is a guide to the proper pronunciation of Sanskrit letters.

अ	*a*	*(but)*
आ	*ā*	*(father)*
इ	*i*	*(it)*
ई	*ī*	*(beat)*
उ	*u*	*(full)*
ऊ	*ū*	*(pool)*
ऋ	*ṛ*	*(rhythm)*
ॠ	*ṝ*	*(marine)*
ऌ	*ḷ*	*(revelry)*
ए	*e*	*(play)*
ऐ	*ai*	*(aisle)*
ओ	*o*	*(go)*
औ	*au*	*(loud)*
क	*ka*	*(seek)* 1
ख	*kha*	*(blockhead)**1
ग	*ga*	*(get)* 1
घ	*gha*	*(log hut)**1
ङ	*ṅa*	*(sing)* 1
च	*ca*	*(chunk)* 2
छ	*cha*	*(catch him)**2
ज	*ja*	*(jump)* 2
झ	*jha*	*(hedgehog)**2
ञ	*ña*	*(bunch)* 2
ट	*ṭa*	*(true)**3
ठ	*ṭha*	*(anthill)**3
ड	*ḍa*	*(drum)**3
ढ	*ḍha*	*(godhead)**3
ण	*ṇa*	*(under)**3
त	*ta*	*(path)**4
थ	*tha*	*(thunder)**4
द	*da*	*(that)**4
ध	*dha*	*(breathe)**4
न	*na*	*(nut)**4
प	*pa*	*(put)* 5
फ	*pha*	*(loophole)**5
ब	*ba*	*(bin)* 5
भ	*bha*	*(abhor)**5
म	*ma*	*(much)* 5
य	*ya*	*(loyal)*
र	*ra*	*(red)*
ल	*la*	*(luck)*
व	*va*	*(vase)*
श	*śa*	*(sure)*
ष	*ṣa*	*(shun)*
स	*sa*	*(so)*
ह	*ha*	*(hum)*

ं	*ṁ*	*anusvāra*	(nasalisation of preceding vowel)
:	*ḥ*	*visarga*	(aspiration of preceding vowel)
*			No exact English equivalents for these letters

1.	Guttural	–	Pronounced from throat
2.	Palatal	–	Pronounced from palate
3.	Lingual	–	Pronounced from cerebrum
4.	Dental	–	Pronounced from teeth
5.	Labial	–	Pronounced from lips

The 5th letter of each of the above class – called nasals – are also pronounced nasally.

Introduction

When one has to interact with the world day after day, stress is to be expected. However, if one can strike a harmony with what one encounters, there is no emotional stress. When one likes what one has to do, then what one does cannot cause any stress. One may like something, but at the same time if it leaves one guilty or sad then one is subject to stress. For instance, a person may love to have alcohol, but in our society there is also a stigma attached to it. Hence, the person taken to alcohol is bound to feel guilty and one's home has no happiness. It will cause stress.

One's interaction with the world being inevitable, stress is a natural consequence. One has to relate to the world for, living is relating to the world. If one can see the difference between being alive and living, I can then say that one need not relate to the world in order to be alive. In sleep, one is alive but one does not relate to anything. So too in coma. In dream, one relates to the objects that one dreams about, without realising they are but projections of oneself.

I relate and therefore there is living. When I am awake, I relate to the world. However, when I relate, either I can strike harmony with what I relate to or I can be the source of disharmony. If the other is a source of disharmony, I can keep myself safe if I have certain space within myself to retain that safety. So, to live a stress-free life, one has to learn that one has the capacity to live in harmony and also one needs to command enough space within to protect oneself from being an emotional victim to others' disturbing actions and behaviour.

The main problem is that it is very difficult to keep the external world external. If I can keep the external things external then I can relate to them, respond to them, objectively, dispassionately. However, more often than not, I allow them to affect me; I internalise situations. If among these three people, Kumar, Mehta and Subbu, I call Kumar, Kumar responds. If I call Mehta, he responds. If I call Subbu, he also responds. If I call out, 'fool,' there is a simultaneous response from all the three. Why? I am just giving you an example to show that we have swallowed a lot and we believe in what we have swallowed. Bhagavān Kṛṣṇa makes a very pertinent statement at the end of the fifth chapter in the *Bhagavad Gītā,*[1] "*sparśān kṛtvā bahir bāhyān…*" It is a very interesting statement that prefaces his talk on meditation in the next chapter, the sixth chapter. He says that one has got to be the meditator first, before one attempts meditation. We are now using meditation for relaxation, but the truth is, the person who is relaxed is the one who is

[1] 5.27

supposed to meditate. One good thing about us is we have our own definitions of meditation and therefore we can all pass!

CLASSICAL DEFINITION OF MEDITATION

The classical definition of meditation is, "*saguṇa-brahma-viṣaya-mānasa-vyāpāraḥ*." Meditation has to be a deliberate mental activity relating to Īśvara, *saguṇaṁ brahma*. Every other action is only a preparation to meditation. The lord gives a preparatory step in these words: *bāhyān sparśān bahiḥ kṛtvā. Spṛśyante iti sparśāḥ*, those people and objects with which you are intimately connected is *sparśa*. Thus, all *sparśa*s are *bāhya*, external. Lord Kṛṣṇa says that keeping all the situations, people and objects external, is imperative to be fit for meditation. You keep them external. The natural question is, 'already they are external; who am I to keep them external?' You cannot externalise something that is already external. But the *Gītā* has definitely something to convey here because even though the people and the objects are external to our senses, some of them can become causes of concern, frustration and so on, making themselves present in our mind; they are inside too.

You can begin the day with this practice: "I visualise a range of mountains, a blue sky, the ocean and the like, things with reference to which I have no demands, I am in harmony with them as they are. I have no agenda for the range of mountains. I have no agenda for the blue sky, nor I have agenda for the trees or the birds. I have no agenda, whatsoever, for all these natural situations and objects."

A COGNITIVE CHANGE WITH REFERENCE TO PEOPLE MAKES ONE A NON-DEMANDING PERSON

With reference to people, in general, perhaps, one can bring oneself to be a non-demanding person. However, when one visualises the significant people in one's life, with whom one is intimately connected, such as one's father, mother, siblings, spouse, children and so on, one cannot take them as objectively as one can take people in general who are not known to one, free from prejudices in terms of colour, race or religion.

I find that it is these significant people who count in my life, whom I cannot take them as they are. I wish they were different. For instance, I may wish my parents to be different in terms of their attitude, behaviour patterns, health and so on. As a child one felt neglected. There is pain, sadness, and anger. These emotions remain in the person as long as they are not processed. Therefore, I have agendas for everyone who is related to me.

Every married person wants the spouse to be a little different. The job of changing each other being incomplete, the marriage is bound to last! Thirty-seven years have passed and they are still trying to change each other. It means that the marriage has not yet begun. It is very typical of married partners. The truth, however, is that nobody can change another person. Lord Kṛṣṇa tried to change Duryodhana and the result was war; Kṛṣṇa could not change Duryodhana.

All that I can do is only try and help another change. If I can bring about a cognitive change in another person, the change in his or her life-style becomes easier.

I can also have agenda for politicians, economists and many others. Consequently, these people are no longer outside; they are inside me. The unfulfilled desires, the demands, the expectations, leave me helpless that turns into frustration. This becomes a permanent source of stress.

There is no stress really speaking, only there is a stressed person. Stress exists only for a structure, a building. A bridge has stress. This body has stress. But I am not discussing that; I am discussing the stressed person, the person who subjects himself or herself to stress. The stressed person is the one who is frustrated, who is not able to live in harmony with one's world. If relating to the world brings stress, I have no way out of stress because I cannot get away from the world in the sense, I cannot stop relating to the world. Of course, I can cut down certain relationships but cutting down relationships would cause stress. I have to relate. Therefore, there is one way out and that is to discover certain space within myself while relating.

I AM DIFFERENT FROM ALL THE ROLES I PLAY

One is called upon to relate to different people, father, mother, son, daughter, spouse, and so on. One has to relate to them. One is son or daughter to one's father. One is son or daughter to one's mother but there is a slight difference. The father's son is different from the mother's son. In relating to different people, one has to play different roles. One plays the role of a husband or wife, father or mother, uncle, cousin, brother, sister, employer, employee, citizen and so on. I use the word, 'role' because one is the same person, who is father and son, mother and daughter. If I am both daughter and mother, it means that I am a daughter with reference to my parents and a mother with reference to my child. Therefore, I am the one who is all these roles. If that is so, then definitely I must be different from any of them. Since I am different from the roles, I can assume the status of any of these. Assumption of a given status is what we can call a role.

THE EXAMPLE OF AN ACTOR AND THE ROLE

Let us look at the example of an actor, A, who plays the role of a beggar B. This actor plays the beggar's role so well that no real life beggar can beg so well as the actor does; the actor has studied and picked up the best nuances of begging. After all, the real life beggar does not have any background music! The actor, therefore, can be the best beggar on the stage. At the same time there is a space within the person. It is that space I am talking of. It is a sacred space, a space that makes the whole role a drama and an enjoyable one, not only for the actor, for the others as well. It is the space of knowledge that is wrought by the awareness that the role is I but I am not the role. When the beggar comes on stage, the actor has to be there. When the beggar talks, the actor talks; the whole anatomy of the beggar is that of the actor. In other words B is A; there is no compromise possible here. Alternative possibility is that B is A, but at the same time, A is not affected by B. He willingly assumed the role of a beggar with the knowledge that he was going to be a beggar. In fact, he accepted the role with the knowledge that he would be richer for being a beggar for an hour or two.

What does that mean? It means there is a self-identity; B is A, but A is not B. It is a different thing altogether. The awareness of the role is the only distance here because between B and A there is no distance—physical, spatial or time-wise. A is not away from B. A is not affected by the miserable, tragic lot of the beggar. According to the script in the play, the beggar suffers a lot of abuse, but Mr. A takes all of them without being in anyway affected. Moreover, according to the script he has to bring tears from his eyes, and he brought a lot of tears rolling down his cheeks. He congratulated himself, "I am crying so well." Not only he felt good, but his friend as well, who was in the audience, who comes to the back stage and congratulates his actor-friend saying, "Hey you cried so well, wonderful! How did you do it?" Thus, he is congratulated for crying. Not only does the actor know that A is free from B, even though B is not free from A, his friend also knows it. The space between A and B is a permanent space. It is the same in real life too.

THE BASIC SIMPLE CONSCIOUS PERSON 'I' IS FREE

A person is given to his or her likes and dislikes, who is ignorant or knowledgeable. When one says one is ignorant, one means that one has knowledge. Why? Because one has that much knowledge to say, "I am ignorant." One is ignorant with reference to what one does not know and is knowledgeable with reference to what one knows. Therefore, one is neither knowledgeable nor ignorant. To say so is a point of view, but a point of view is not the view. Therefore, it is very evident that one is either ignorant or knowledgeable with reference to what one knows or does not know. Similarly, I am a liker with reference to what I like; with reference to what I do not like, I am a disliker. It means I am neither liker nor a disliker.

EVERY ROLE IS FRAUGHT WITH CHALLENGES

Everyday I wear so many hats; play so many roles, but the basic person is me. Role-playing can be very tiresome and stressful if there is no space while playing the role for no role is free of difficulty or obstacle, either in real life or on stage.

Every role, be it the role of a father, the mother, a son, a daughter and so on, is not going to be without problems. The role of mother is not going to be without some challenges, especially these days. Even though the child is only two-year old or three-year old, the parents have to get admission in a nursery school. It is a big thing. The parents have to get letter of recommendation. It is just ridiculous but that is how it is. As a mother you have challenges. In fact every role has challenges. All these challenges turn into frustrations if they are not met with, and thereby leading to stress.

Therefore, I say that there is a basic person that is you, a conscious person, a relaxed person. To see this fact, it does not take time; it takes attention. It takes insight.

This is what you are, the basic person, a conscious being. The basic person is not the willing person.

With the eyes open you are seer, with ears open you are a hearer; in other words, you are a simple conscious person. It is this conscious person who becomes a thinker, a seer, a hearer, liker, disliker, walker, talker, father, mother, and so on. One can play any number of roles with their relevant scripts to follow, if only one cares to know and pay attention to the fact that, 'I am a simple conscious person.'

There can be no contention to this that one is a simple conscious person and that person is free. The person is not the role, but the role is the person. When one does not see this, there is confusion; both the role and the person are rolled into one. Further, since the role is fraught with challenges one cannot avoid stress. B is A, A is not B and the A is I.

GIVING OTHERS FREEDOM TO BE WHAT THEY ARE

You can avoid stress by keeping all the people outside by granting them the freedom to be what they are. Let the father be the father in your kindness and love. Grant the person the freedom to be what he is. Every person can be whatever that person is because each person has a background, a family background, a social background, a cultural background, and so on, that accounts for the person's behaviour. However disconcerting it may be, however unbecoming of the person it may be, but still it is in the background of the person who needs help.

UNDERSTANDING KEEPS ONE AWAY FROM STRESS

You can be very understanding, but that does not mean that you have to allow yourself to be trampled upon by others. You draw a line between yourself and the person you need to deal with. You have a threshold of tolerance. In terms of giving, in terms of time, in terms of everything, you have a threshold. You draw a line and you operate within the line. You do not allow yourself or the other person to cross the line. You can always tell the person that you are sorry that you cannot handle this as equipped as you want to. You can kindly point out without evoking the defence mechanism in the other.

You have to learn to keep away from stress. In fact you have to live an alert life. You have to grant the freedom to everyone who is intimately related to you. You find in yourself enough space to have compassion. There is love. When these are there, you will find there is no room for stress at all. I am talking of emotional stress. Physical stress is inevitable.

Emotional stress is the problem that we want to deal with here. By dealing with emotional stress, perhaps, the other stress also we may reduce.

RELATING IS ENJOYABLE WHEN YOU GRANT FREEDOM TO OTHERS TO BE WHAT THEY ARE

You have to grant freedom to the people to be what they are. In one sentence I say, in a relationship, you are as free in that relationship as the freedom you grant to the other. Think it over. The more freedom you give to the other, the freer you are in the relationship. You do not need freedom from the relationship. If you need freedom from one relationship, you will get related to another, again needing freedom from that relationship, because there is a basic problem.

You need to relate anyway, since relating is living. You need freedom in relationship and that freedom is always in the offing. It is never yours until you learn to grant freedom to the other to be what that person is. If you grant that freedom, perhaps you can help the person change because there is no tension. If you want to change the other without understanding the person, the attempts will be construed as offensive.

Relating to a person is enjoyable only when you grant freedom to that person to be as he or she is, as long as that person does not cross the *lakṣmaṇa-rekhā*, the boundary line, that you have drawn. You have to safeguard that. You have no reason to be free from relationship when you can find freedom in relationship. Understanding the advice of the *Gītā*,[2] "keeping the external objects external..." is important.

Keeping the external things, external. Suppose, you buy a ticket to travel, to be away from people, do you know there are many stowaways who are travelling along with you? They are the very persons you want to get away from. The fact that they bother you travels with you. Along with the fact, the constituents of the fact also would travel with you. They are in your mind, travelling with you without tickets!

---

[2] *sparśān kṛtvā bahir bāhyān...* (*Bhagavadgītā* 5.27)

LIFE IS A SERIES OF DECISIONS

As an individual I have to make decisions. I find the most difficult thing to do in life is to make decision, sometimes, painful decisions. You are your decisions.

The *gāyatrī-mantra*, that an eight-year old child is initiated into, has this excellent prayer. Initially it serves as a prayer even though there is so much in the *mantra* to be understood. The *mantra* says, "*yaḥ bargaḥ naḥ (asmākaṁ) dhiyaḥ (buddhayaḥ) pracodayāt (pracodanaṁ kuryāt)*." May that Lord abiding in my heart, who is all-knowledge, free from ignorance, like the sun who is free from darkness, brighten my mind to the ways of thinking that would make me decide properly. May he set our minds on the right way of thinking leading to clear decisions.

Your life is your decisions, a series of decisions, which have made you what you are today. It is not always possible to be at the right place at the right time. Therefore, the prayer is, "May I decide properly to be at the right place at the right time." Really this is the most comprehensive prayer in one line.

PROCRASTINATION IS A SOURCE OF STRESS

You have to decide without procrastination. You can postpone, but procrastination is a habit that causes stress. If you decide to postpone deciding, that is totally acceptable. You are angry now and you have to decide. You decide not to decide. That is a prudent decision. In anger even if you decide, do not execute that decision. Keep it pending. You write a letter, but do not post it. When you are calm, again write it. May be writing in anger is good; acting upon it is certainly not. Understand; do not post that letter.

Deliberate postponement is not a cause for stress. But procrastination, yes. You keep procrastinating, "I will do it tomorrow. I will do it tomorrow." The files on the table keep piling up. Later they go to the drawer. This is the reason why the drawers are provided in your table! When the files are on the table, the sight of them makes you guilty. Hence, you push them inside the drawer so that the tabletop is always clean. But you cannot hide the knowledge that there are files to be disposed off; they are always in your mind, causing stress. Therefore, procrastination does not help.

In decision-making, do the most painful thing first. You can do the pleasant things later. Someone said, "Swamiji, I listen to your talks on procrastination. It is wonderful; I am going to follow this from next week." (Laughter). This is a typical procrastinator. One will lose relationships, friendships; one will lose one's job perhaps. Procrastination is the worst cause of stress.

Handling helpless situations

We have to act upon a helpless situation. In today's world of Internet and e-mail, we are, more often than before, led into situations where we are helpless. We want the politicians to be above corruption, but I hear from some intelligent people that this is not an issue anymore! These people are shameless, absolutely shameless. Corruption is an issue. It is the only issue. Every other issue issues from this. If this issue is settled, we can address all issues with planning. Otherwise all plans get derailed. That the leaders of our country are corrupt makes us helpless. Stress follows. The daily tabloids with huge letters shock us with items of news, day after day making us feel helpless. Stress. Thus, there are many helpless situations—economic, familial, domestic and so on.

Stress disappears when you act upon a helpless situation

If you remain in a helpless state, there would be stress. When you act upon it, helplessness disappears. That is why you have got letters-to-the-editor columns in the daily newspapers. You write a letter to the editor and feel that you have done something. It is a stress-releasing action. (Laughter). Another thing you can do. You can write whatever you want to write on the Internet. At least, those who want to read will read. (Laughter). A third option is that you can pray. Pray for the person who says, 'corruption is not an issue.' Pray for that person. Then, you are not helpless because you have acted, seeking help. Prayer is an action.

How to handle an argument

People have different kinds of perceptions of a given fact. Sometimes, these become causes for an argument. Dissimilar likes and dislikes are inevitable because two minds never think alike. They do influence our perceptions of any given situation. We can command objectively, in our perception, when we are not influenced by our likes and dislikes, and being influenced by them we are subjective. However, the person who is subjective is totally unaware of his or her own subjectivity. That kind of clash in perceptions in a dialogue ends up in heated arguments.

In an argument it is very fundamental to know whether the topic of discussion is relative. For instance, one can argue whether the Republican or the Democratic Party is good. On this issue one can argue on both sides and the one who can argue tactfully will always silence the other; there is no victory!

On the other hand, in a discussion there is no final winner because a discussion is meant for revealing the facts. Discussion is helpful and it is also healthy. Moreover, through discussion one is likely to look at the situation differently and therefore one can have better objectivity.

In an argument one is obsessed with one's own stand and ideas about a particular fact, whereas in a discussion one can see the other side properly. In a discussion there is no victory for anyone; there is only understanding.

In Sanskrit, an argument is called '*jalpa,*' where the attempt is only to win and never to accept the defeat. That is why arguments are never healthy, while discussions are. An argument can create problems; like when you lose your temper and say undesirable things. When you are in a tight corner in an argument, it is easier to get angry and become defensive. Like they say, "The best form of defense is offense." Even before an argument begins you launch an offensive attack on the person, a kind of pre-emptive strike. You punch the fellow before he punches you because, if he punches you first, he may not stick around when it is your turn to punch him. Accordingly, you may adopt the same policy in an argument where there is no real discussion.

It is not always possible to avoid an argument. For instance, in an earthquake if the tremors are not small, then there will be a huge eruption. So, it is only to avoid big outbursts I say, small arguments are better; it helps you, at least, to ease the tension. But, if you avoid these small arguments, they will eventually blow up. When you are confronted with an argument and even though you choose not to argue, the anger will be bottled up inside. Sooner or later this bottled up anger explodes. The explosion may be on a very petty topic like, "There is no salt in this food." The explosions that follow are not caused by the absence of adequate salt—that was only a trigger for the emotions to come out.

Vedanta does not advocate avoiding an argument. In fact, the very teaching of Vedanta is through discussions. A student raises an objection or the *śāstra* itself raises one and that is clarified with an explanation. It is an excellent way of analysing and understanding the truth of a topic. This process of raising an objection and getting clarification is possible only in a discussion, where you make sure all issues are settled.

ARGUMENTS ARE INTRINSIC TO NEGATIVE EMOTIONS

Let us look at another point that deals with the emotional predicament. Most of the arguments involve intense emotional situations leading to a personal attack and losing sight of the issue to be resolved.

When one cannot avoid an argument due to the differences in one's likes and dislikes, one is then setting oneself up for a no-win situation. Take for instance, a couple together go for shopping. One does not like what the other one wants to buy. Soon it becomes very personal. "You have this habit," one says; "not only you, your mother also has the same habit," the other goes on and on. Thus, an argument begins over a trivial choice of a shade of colour which is no longer the issue discussed!

There are certain realities we need to understand; they are not open to options. One plus one is two for all. Likes and dislikes have no role to play in knowing. Understanding our emotions also calls for objectivity.

People come from varied backgrounds. Background includes one's parentage, economic, political and social environment, religion and culture. The person's background builds the core personality that may have many issues to process. It is not enough that you accept your background; you need to accept others' background as well. This acceptance makes you objective in spite of your background. In other words, to be objective in your perception you need to accept what you are, accept your own subjectivity. That helps you accept others' subjectivity too. There is sympathy, understanding, and healthy dialogue.

In a healthy dialogue you can say what you feel, but with an honest acknowledgement that you may be wrong: "This is how I see, I may be wrong." When you say this sentence, please mean it and you will see it works; it will help you avoid an argument!

UNDERSTANDING WHAT IS LAKṢMĪ

Please understand Lakṣmī is not just money. You will lose your domestic happiness, Gṛhalakṣmī, because you think Lakṣmī is only money, Dhanalakṣmī. In Chennai, on the beach, there is a temple dedicated to different forms of Lakṣmī.

A good home gives you domestic happiness. To make a home you need to be available at home. You have to be a welcome person at home. The members of your family should never get prepared with fastened seat belts for your arrival! You should not be looked upon as a source of terror. Let them welcome you with eagerness. For that you have to spend time with your children because there is Santānalakṣmī, wealth of children. Make the spouse happy because she is Varalakṣmī, wealth of marital happiness.

Trust in the goodness of people, in the laws that govern, in their legitimacy, in their correctness, and so on and it will give you Dhairayalakṣmī, wealth of courage.

It is not at all possible to fulfil all your desires. But if you can manage your desires, then there is also Jayalakṣmī in your life, wealth of the capacity to manage. Now, your life is free from stress because you have taken care of everything to avoid stress. All forms of Lakṣmī being there, life is filled with meaning and doing.

Guided Meditation

Human free will finds its total expression in voluntary prayers. In prayerful moments, one is totally with oneself. This is a blessing.

The past seems to have a tight hold on each of us. To let go one's past is not in the hands of one's will. If one can have a degree of awareness of this problem, one can discover hope and solution in a well-directed prayer or guided meditation.

Meditation is an act invoking grace as well as a simple autosuggestion. As I sit in meditation, relaxed, I offer a prayer to the Lord whom I invoke in any given form, in any given name.

These few pages bring to you some of the meditation-prayers I conducted for my disciples in the *gurukula*. When you read them, be with the words and keep seeing their meaning.

I mentally Pray:

O Lord, I cannot change

my childhood...

my parentage, my entire past...

What has happened in my life
I cannot change...
What has happened
has happened...
I cannot do anything about it...

On the basis of what has happened
I am not sad or angry...
I accept gracefully
whatever has happened in my life...

There are a lot of things
that I can change...
that I can repair...

I seek the strength of will
and the ability
to make proper, adequate efforts...
to change...

I do not waste my time
trying to change
what I cannot change...

Nor do I want to waste my time
putting up with unhealthy situations
that I can change...

The difference between the two...
what I can
and cannot change
is not easy to distinguish...
It takes wisdom
for which I again invoke your grace...

O Lord
May I have the maturity
to accept gracefully
what I cannot change...
The will and effort...
to change
what I can...
And the wisdom
to know the difference...

I am just awake
alive to what happens

at this moment...
I lay down
my will...
my choice...

I am just awake
to the moment...
Moment to moment...
my being aware of the moment
does not fluctuate...

My being aware
of the moment
is an abiding
lasting ever-present fact...

My being aware
is not in fits and starts...
It is a presence...
a presence which is always present.

Oṁ tat sat

Books by Swami Dayananda Saraswati

Public Talk Series :

1. Living Intelligently
2. Successful Living
3. Need for Cognitive Change
4. Discovering Love
5. The Value of Values
6. Vedic View and Way of Life

Upaniṣad Series :

7. Muṇḍakopaniṣad
8. Kenopaniṣad

Prakaraṇa Series :

9. Tattvabodhaḥ

Text Translation Series :

10. Śrīmad Bhagavad Gītā
    (Text with roman transliteration and English translation)
11. Śrī Rudram
    (Text in Sanskrit with transliteration, word-to-word and verse meaning along with an elaborate commentary in English)

Stotra Series :

12. Dīpārādhanā
13. Prayer Guide
    (With explanations of several Mantras, Stotras, Kirtans and Religious Festivals)

Moments with Oneself Series :

14. Freedom from Helplessness
15. Living versus Getting On
16. Insights
17. Action and Reaction
18. Fundamental Problem
19. Problem is You, Solution is You
20. Purpose of Prayer
21. Vedanta 24x7
22. Freedom
23. Crisis Management
24. Surrender and Freedom
25. The Need for Personal Reorganisation
26. Freedom in Relationship
27. Stress-free Living
28. Om Namo Bhagavate Vāsudevāya
29. Yoga of Objectivity

Bhagavad Gītā

30. Bhagavad Gītā Home Study Course (Hardbound - 9 Volumes)

Meditation Series :

31. Morning Meditation Prayers
32. What is Meditation?

Essays :

33. Do all Religions have the same goal?
34. Conversion is Violence
35. Gurupūrṇimā
36. Dānam
37. Japa
38. Can We?
39. Moments with Krishna
40. Teaching Tradition of Advaita Vedanta
41. Compositions of Swami Dayananda Saraswati

Exploring Vedanta Series : (*vākyavicāra*)

42. śraddhā bhakti dhyāna yogād avaihi ātmānaṁ ced vijānīyāt

Books translated in other languages and in English based on Swami Dayananda Saraswati's Original Exposition

Tamil

43. Veeduthorum Gitopadesam (9 Volumes)
    (Bhagavad Gītā Home Study Course)
44. Dānam

Kannada

45. Mane maneyalli Adhyayana (7 Volumes)
(Bhagavad Gītā Home Study Course)
46. Vedanta Pravesike

Malayalam

47. Muṇḍakopaniṣad

Hindi

48. Ghar baithe Gītā Vivecan (Vol 1)
(Bhagavad Gītā Home Study Course)
49. Antardṛṣṭi (Insights)
50. Vedanta 24X7
51. Kriya aur Pratikriya (Action and Reaction)

English

52. The Jungian Myth and Advaita Vedanta
53. The Vedantic Self and the Jungian Psyche
54. Salutations to Rudra
55. Without a Second

Biography

56. Swami Dayananda Saraswati
Contributions & Writings
(Smt. Sheela Balalji)

Distributed in India & worldwide by

MOTILAL BANARSIDASS - NEW DELHI

Tel : 011 - 2385 8335 / 2385 1985 / 2385 2747

Also available at :

ARSHA VIDYA RESEARCH AND PUBLICATION TRUST
32 / 4 Sir Desika Road
Mylapore Chennai 600 004
Telefax : 044 - 2499 7131
Email : avrandpc@gmail.com
Website : www.avrpt.com

ARSHA VIDYA GURUKULAM
Anaikatti P.O.
Coimbatore 641 108
Ph : 0422 - 2657001
Fax : 0422 - 2657002
Email : office@arshavidya.in
Website : www.arshavidya.in

ARSHA VIDYA GURUKULAM
P.O.Box 1059. Pennsylvania
PA 18353, USA
Ph : 001-570-992-2339
Email : avp@epix.net
Website : www.arshavidya.org

SWAMI DAYANANDA ASHRAM
Purani Jhadi, P.B.No. 30
Rishikesh, Uttaranchal 249 201
Telefax: 0135 - 2430769
Email : ashrambookstore@yahoo.com
Website : www.dayananda.org

Other leading Book Stores:

Chennai:	**044**
Motilal Banarsidass	2498 2315
Giri Trading	2495 1966
Higginbothams	2851 3519
Pustak Bharati	2461 1345
Theosophical Publishing House	2446 6613 / 2491 1338
The Odessey	43910300

Bengaluru:		**080**
	Gangarams	2558 1617 / 2558 1618
	Sapna Book House	4011 4455 / 4045 5999
	Strand Bookstall	2558 2222, 2558 0000
	Vedanta Book House	2650 7590
Coimbatore:		**0422**
	Guru Smruti	9486773793
	Giri Trading	2541523
Trivandrum:		**0471**
	Prabhus Bookhouse	2478397 / 2473496
Kozhikode:		**0471**
	Ganga Bookhouse	6521262
Mumbai:		**022**
	Chetana Bookhouse	2285 1243 / 2285 3412
	Strand Bookstall	2266 1994 / 2266 1719/ 2261 4613
	Giri Trading	2414 3140